Tourette Syndrome:

What Families Should Know

By

Elaine Fantle Shimberg

Dedicated
to the memory of
Arthur K. Shapiro, M.D.

Acknowledgments

This book was the inspiration of the Tourette Syndrome Association's President, Judit Ungar, who requested a book addressing what families wanted to know about TS. I was happy to do so as a "thank you" for all the advice and support my family and I have received from that amazing organization over the years.

I could not have written it without great input from many families, including members of my own family, all of whom have experienced living with Tourette Syndrome.

Special thanks to Gary Frank, Sue Levi-Pearl, and others from the Tourette Syndrome Association, who spent long hours reading my manuscript with red pen in hand to make certain that it was accurate in every way; to Veronica Tillis, my favorite proofreader, to Kathy Zimmerman, Kasey Kelly and to Sandy Walling at Abernathy House Publishing who turned the manuscript into a beautiful book.

OTHER BOOKS BY
ELAINE FANTLE SHIMBERG

The Complete Single Father (co-authored)

Helga, the Hippotamouse (children's book)

Herman, the Hermit Crab (children's book)

Another Chance for Love (co-authored)

Coping with COPD: Chronic Obstructive Pulmonary Disease

*Coping with Chronic Heartburn: What You Need to Know
    About Acid Reflux and GERD*

*Blending Families: A Guide for Parents, Stepparents, and
Everyone Building a Successful New Family*

Write Where You Live

How to Get Out of the Hospital Alive (co-authored)

A Heritage of Helping: Shriners' Hospitals

Living with Tourette Syndrome

Gifts of Time (co-authored)

Depression: What Families Should Know

Strokes: What Families Should Know

Relief from IBS: Irritable Bowel Syndrome

Coping with Kids and Vacation (co-authored)

*Two for the Money: A Woman's Guide to a Double Career
    Marriage* (co-authored)

How to Be a successful Housewife/Writer

INTRODUCTION

Who am I to write a book on *Tourette Syndrome: What Families Should Know?* I'm not a physician, nor psychologist, nor nurse, nor scientist.

I am, however, a medical writer, but more importantly, I not only have Tourette Syndrome myself, but three of my five children (now adults) have Tourette Syndrome. (Needless to say, my husband and I watch our twelve grandchildren carefully for any sign of a potential tic that could signify that one or more of them may have inherited that genetic trait.)

My adult children with TS and I now, have mild, if any symptoms, other than an occasional neck jerk or blink when we get stressed or fatigued. The word "now," however, is the operative word, because we had no diagnosis for the first child for five years, until she was twelve. I lost track of how many neurologists, allergists, and psychologists we dragged her to looking for answers. (When she was finally diagnosed correctly, that's when I also learned that my "habits" were really Tourette Syndrome tics.) Until that time, my husband and I were told that the kids were neurotic, I was neurotic, the kids were emotionally disturbed, I was emotionally disturbed, I was a bad parent, etc.

We experienced the same frustration as many of you have—well-meaning suggestions from family and friends, disbelief from teachers and coaches, confusing medical advice from uninformed physicians who called it the "cursing disease," and heartbreak as our kids were teased by their peers.

Fortunately, thanks to the efforts of the Tourette Syndrome Association (TSA) and its dedicated professional and lay volunteers, a larger proportion of the medical community and lay population today has at least heard of TS and more individuals are now aware that TS is a chronic neurobiological disorder consisting of both motor and vocal tics that come and go over a period of time. It is not a psychological disorder, an "acting out" of resentments, a nervous habit, nor a means of getting attention.

The tics are "unvoluntary," not involuntary, because the individual can usually hold them back for a short time, but eventually, they must be expressed, like a sneeze. Therefore, it is difficult and exhausting to continually try to mask the symptoms. For that and other reasons, TS does affect an entire family. The more everyone in your family circle (along with close friends and co-workers) understand what TS is and isn't, the lower the stress level and the easier life will be, especially for the person with TS.

How do you get others to understand about TS?

You educate them.

Table of Contents

PART I: After the Diagnosis

Chapter 1: *Responding to the Diagnosis*

Chapter 2: *Overcoming Guilt*

Chapter 3: *Educating Family, Friends, and Others*

Chapter 4: *Understanding School Issues*

PART II: It's All in the Family

Chapter 5: *Coping with Sibling Reactions*

Chapter 6: *Deciphering Tics from Behavioral Issues*

Chapter 7: *Balancing Tics and Treatment*

Chapter 8: *Recognizing Related Disorders*

Chapter 9: *Knowing What TS Isn't*

Chapter 10: *Reducing Stress*

PART III: Adult Issues

Chapter 11: *Getting a Job*

Chapter 12: *Dating (for adults with TS)*

Chapter 13: *Securing Housing*

Chapter 14: *Looking into the Future*

Resources

Suggested Reading

Index

Part One:

After the Diagnosis

Chapter 1

Responding to the Diagnosis

Parental reactions differ greatly when a child is diagnosed with Tourette Syndrome. For some (including my husband and me), it was a great relief to know that our child was not mentally ill or trying to get attention and that the disorder, although unpredictable and frustrating, was not life threatening.

Others, however, admit that the diagnosis is a tremendous emotional blow, as they realized that their dream of having the "perfect" child, is destroyed. One mother told me bitterly, "I wish I hadn't learned that there really was something wrong. I was fine while I was still in denial." For these parents, there is a very real sense of grief and true mourning. Parents like these are frightened, a fear triggered, in part, by many myths perpetuated by the media along with its examples of the worst case scenarios.

I was recently approached by a network program that wanted to have me and my three adult kids with TS on their show. When I explained that their tics were hardly noticeable, they backed off. "But it's a wonderful encouragement for others with TS," I said. They disagreed, saying "TV is a visual medium. We want to show when it's bad, not good."

Many parents drive themselves crazy trying to make sense of things by questioning what they must have done wrong. "Was it that glass of wine during pregnancy?" "Could it have been triggered by having another child too soon?" "Could I have caused it in some way and if so, how?" "Is it something from your side of the family or mine? And if so, who?"

How Family Dynamics May Change

It isn't unusual for one parent to have a more difficult time adjusting to the diagnosis than the other, regardless of whether they are married or divorced. This can create misunderstandings and tension between the parents, just at a time when they need to comfort one another and work as a team for their child. When parents battle a diagnosis, they cause more stress for their entire family, especially the youngster who is also struggling to accept the diagnosis and this added stress tends to make the tics worse.

Force yourselves to talk freely and honestly about your feelings and listen to what your partner is saying (and not saying). It's understandable how one or both parents may refuse to accept the diagnosis, especially as the TS symptoms tend to wax and wane, that is, they get worse and then better. It's tempting to say, "It's just a nervous habit. It will go away, just like last time" or, "You see? He isn't making that barking sound anymore."

Whatever the reaction, it's universal that family dynamics change when there is a child with a chronic illness. It not only affects the parents, but also the siblings, if any, the grandparents, and the other relatives. As I wrote in my previous book, *Living with Tourette Syndrome*, "Needs, expectations, and responsibilities are all altered, sometimes subtly, occasionally rather dramatically."

It's important to realize that the family's reaction to the diagnosis of TS and the quality of the support the family offers can greatly affect the child's development, influencing it either positively or negatively. Hopefully, the information contained in this book will help guide parents and the entire family in a manner that will minimize emotional and physical trauma and help to preserve a youngster's delicate self-esteem.

Chapter 2

Overcoming Guilt

There's no use simply saying, "Don't feel guilty," because most parents do. If there's anything wrong with our kids, it's human to feel that it's our fault and to assume the blame. "I let him go to school without a jacket and that's why he has pneumonia." "I made too many desserts and that's why she has diabetes." "My grandfather blinked a lot so the tics must have come from my side of the family." "Why am I being punished by God?"

Even when you can accept the reality that your child has a chronic disorder called Tourette Syndrome (TS), often there's also a sense of guilt because you and your spouse fussed at your child whenever he/she made vocalizations or had motor tics. You tried bribes to stop the tics or at least, make them less noticeable. You may have even spanked or otherwise punished your youngster. But now that you have a diagnosis and know that your youngster can't control the sounds or movements, you may feel even more guilty.

You may feel guilty because you or another family member has TS and you know that in most cases, TS is genetically transmitted. Try to think about it rationally. Would you have preferred not having your child because he/she has TS? Of course not. Remember that you also may have passed along some wonderful genetic traits— beautiful skin, curly hair, perfect teeth, an ability to handle numbers, play music, perform on the stage, throw a perfect pass, etc.

Be Kind to Yourself; You're Human

What can you do? Remember that you're a human being, not a perfect entity. Forgive yourself, release your sense of feeling guilty, and go on with your life. Learn all you can about TS, but also remember that it is your child's disorder, not yours. He/she will have to live life and cope with the tics especially when they occur at inopportune times, learn to handle questions and/or teasing, and make necessary adjustments to help in school, work, social life, etc.

You and the rest of the family will have to perfect a delicate balancing act. Support the child, but don't hover. Your child needs to have control and know that you think he/she is a capable individual. When you try to live your child's life, you are saying, in essence, "We don't trust you to handle this." So the youngster may stop trying.

What if you feel guilty about being so stressed from the constant hooting, sniffing, or barking, those vocal tics that seemingly never let up? It's exhausting to hear them, no doubt, but it's also draining to the person with the vocal tics who can't get away from them. But you can.

Accept that it's normal to sometimes want to get away from the sounds and sights of the tics. That doesn't mean you don't want to be around your child, it's just that you need some time away from the symptoms. Don't feel guilty about that either, as we've all felt that way from time to time. So go out for dinner occasionally for a "date night" without the kids, play golf or bridge, jog or swim, or whatever works to give yourself a break.

Spend some time with your friends as well. Don't hide the fact that your child has TS. There's nothing to be ashamed of, no more than if he/she had diabetes or wore glasses. You'll not only be educating them about TS, but you're **encouraging** them to become more patient and understanding when your youngster is around.

If you get stuck in this "I feel so guilty" mode, counseling from a professional therapist may be helpful.

Chapter 3

Educating Family, Friends, and Others

You may find that some folks just "don't get it." Friends and relatives may suggest that you just need to be more firm with your child and he/she will stop "doing those things to get attention." Explain that your child would love to stop making the hoots, yelps, and sniffs or jerking his/her neck, blinking, or numerous other motor actions, but it's part of the neurological disorder called Tourette Syndrome. And no, cutting his hair won't keep your son from jerking his head and the constant sniffing isn't from allergies; it's caused by this neurological disorder called Tourette Syndrome. Explain that while it's true that your child might be able to control the tics for a time, eventually the tics must be expressed, like a sneeze.

How to Educate Others
There are many ways for you to share what you've learned about TS with others. The Tourette Syndrome Association, Inc. has numerous pamphlets and videos that are yours for the asking, many for minimal cost or without charge or posted on the TSA web site. I've written a number of them…including *When Your Grandchild Has TS*; *Dear Diary, My Sibling Has TS*; *Divorce, Tourette Syndrome, and the Family*; and *Coping with Tourette Syndrome: A Parent's Viewpoint*. But there are

17

other excellent ones for you to get for your child's school, including *The Educator's Guide; What School Bus Drivers Need to Know About TS; TS in the Classroom;, TS and the School Nurse*, etc. A complete list of suggested reading is in the back of this book.

There also are video tapes and DVDs available online at the Tourette Syndrome Association web site. One of the most recent is the Emmy Award-winning, "I Have Tourette's, But Tourette's Doesn't Have Me."

NOTE: Be careful about what you read online. Many web sites contain incorrect information or describe only the experience of one particular individual, often one who has a severe case of TS or who also has what I call "tag along conditions," like OCD, anxiety, learning disabilities, ADD, disruptive behavior, etc.

TS is a spectrum disorder. That means there are many people with mild symptoms at one end and then there are others who have severe symptoms. In fact, the Tourette Syndrome Association, Inc. (TSA) theorizes that there are many people with mild symptoms who never see a doctor about them. Although my adult children with TS had more severe symptoms when they were younger (from about ages 9-15), they now have very mild or often unnoticeable tics. For accurate information, focus on the Tourette Syndrome Association's web site (www.tsa-usa..org) or those provided by leading medical centers.

It's important that you and your entire family become an advocate for your child, for your child's sake so you can help those around him to be supportive. Tourette Syndrome can appear to be a strange disorder, sometimes even a little frightening for people who don't understand what it is. Susan Conners, an educator and long time advocate for TS, a disorder she herself experiences first hand, says, "TS is not fatal. Children don't die from TS, but their spirits are killed every day because of society's reaction to their symptoms and the treatment they receive."

Grandparents Can Provide a Safe Harbor

Lucky is the child with supportive grandparents, especially if that child has Tourette Syndrome. As I wrote in my book, *Blending Families*, "Grandparents are the great equalizer in a child's life; they are the strong safety in the 'them versus us' game, which (often) pairs grandparent and grandchild against the parents. Mindful of their own child-rearing errors (and acutely aware of those being made daily by their adult child), grandparents become a safe harbor when the sailing gets rough. It offers one that rarity in life---a second chance."

At first, it may not always be easy to educate your parents (or those of your spouse) about Tourette Syndrome. They may be convinced in the beginning that the tics are the result of your lack of discipline, the fact that you both work outside the home, that you have too many kids (or only the one), or a myriad of other judgment calls, based in part because they don't want to believe that their beloved grandchild could really have a chronic condition that's causing this type of unusual behavior.

Once they understand, however, (thanks to the educational materials available from the TSA), they probably will become their grandchild's fiercest defender. Grandparents can become the child's confidant, give parents a breather by taking the youngster overnight or out for ice cream, or just offer that special one-on-one time that most parents find in such short supply, especially when they have other children as well. Grandparents plant the seed of self-esteem in their grandchildren, water it with unconditional love, and then delight as it grows.

Chapter 4

Understanding School Issues

Once your child has been diagnosed with TS, you probably worked hard with the teacher, explaining what TS is and isn't and offering videos and other educational information. But remember that as your child advances from class to class, your work is far from done as you also need to help educate the next group of teachers. You're not just clearing a more comfortable path for your own child, but also for other children who travel the same way.

School, for any child who is "different," is a struggle. (It doesn't matter if the youngster has TS, is shorter than peers, is obese, has learning disabilities, ADHD, OCD, is dyslexic, stutters, limps, wears glasses, or has any number of other differences. The child who's "different" is prey to bullies and others who tease and taunt in order to boost their own lack of self-esteem.) The child with TS, however, may also have a variety of these additional difficulties along with impulsive behavior, vocal and physical tics, some of which could become potentially harmful to the other students, such as an arm jerking when the child with TS has scissors in her hand, or inadvertently tripping someone when the child has a leg tic.

That's why it's so vital to have frequent educational sessions with teachers, school nurses, coaches, bus drivers, and other school personnel, so they understand TS and its various expressions, and can help a youngster with TS cope with

20

psycho-social problems related to the disorder as well as create ways in which learning may become more productive.

If your youngster is comfortable with the idea, give the teacher permission to pass along the knowledge to the class to alleviate any fears the children may have. They can learn that TS isn't catching, that no one dies from it, and having it doesn't mean you're crazy. If your child is willing to be in the classroom at this time, she may want to answer questions the classmates may have.

Remember that it's unlikely that your child is the only one in the class with special needs. One year, a teacher had one of my children with TS, another with hemophilia, another who was hearing impaired, and another with epilepsy. My guess is that she also had a few with learning disabilities and ADHD. Because she was a caring teacher, the children learned a great deal about tolerance and focusing on each other's strong points, along with spelling, math, and history.

Always be tactful when dealing with your child's teachers or principal. Don't be antagonistic, angry, or defensive, regardless of how frustrated you may feel. Smile. Your child is only one of probably thirty in the class. Most teachers do try to do their best, while also dealing with required testing, lack of supplies, and often poor pay for very hard, yet extremely important work—educating our kids.

Work with them, treat them with respect, and try to help whenever possible, by being a homeroom parent, tutoring other kids, and attending parent-teacher conferences. (Note: Even if you're divorced, go as a team for the sake of your child and the over-worked teacher who doesn't want to have to schedule separate conferences just because the two of you do not wish to be together in the same room for your child's benefit).

Know Your Legal Rights

First of all, it's important to know that you have legal rights concerning your child's education. The "Individuals with Disabilities Education Act" (IDEA), or Public Law 101-476 states that "children with disabilities who are demonstrating significant difficulty in their school and/or academic performance are guaranteed a free and appropriate public education." If a school system can't provide this, they must explore other options and, in some cases, pay for something that works. Since 2006, as a result of TSA's advocacy efforts, TS has been included in the "Other Health Impaired" (OHI) category of the IDEA, which means it is the official classification for youngsters with TS in every school throughout the United States.

Once it is determined that your child qualifies, you and the school officials meet to decide which, if any, accommodations should be made in order for your child to succeed.

Learn to Speak the Academics' Language

Every profession has its own special language, but if you're going to be your child's advocate, you need to learn that lexicon…and quickly. Educators, like hospital personnel, speak in acronyms and assume you understand. When you don't…and that may occur frequently at first, ask for a translation. Don't just nod your head for fear that if you ask, they'll think you're stupid. Here's a partial crib sheet so you'll be prepared:

- IEP means "individualized education plan." It is the plan that you and the school will agree upon and may include your child being tested orally, rather than with a written test; using a typewriter, if the handwriting is illegible; and being permitted to leave the classroom if a severe tic is frequent in order to express it in private.
- LD means "learning disabled."

- SED means "socially or emotionally disturbed."
- Mainstreaming means placing children with disabilities in the regular classroom.
- "On task" simply means that your youngster is working and not staring into space, doodling, fidgeting, etc.

Out of the Mouths of Babes

Once your child understands more about TS and feels comfortable talking about it, he/she can turn lemons into lemonade. Many school-age children with TS have turned their disorder into a winning science project by telling classmates about their experiences with TS. Usually, their peers are fascinated and even those who may have teased in the past, change their behavior. But don't force your child to talk about it if he/she feels uncomfortable or embarrassed. Protect your child's self-esteem at all times. It's very fragile.

How to Help the Teachers Teach

A growing number of internationally-known special education teachers and psychologists, including Susan Conners, M.Ed.; Jacqueline Favish, M.Ed., Harvey C. Parker, Ph.D., and Ramona Fisher-Collins, M.Ed., have tested and shared a number of specific accommodations that can be helpful to children with TS, as well as ADD and OCD and also helpful for their teachers. Many of them are found on the education page on TSA's web site at www.tsa-usa.org. You might suggest the following to your child's teachers:

- **For inattention, use side-front seating.**

   While it's natural for teachers to seat children who are inattentive in the center front row, that's one of the worst places for children with TS to sit because they know that everyone behind them can see their tics. They try harder to withhold the tics, which creates even more stress and ultimately, makes the tics even worse and interferes with their concentration.

- **Establish private "stay on task" cues**
  Rather than singling out the child with TS and reminding him to stay on task, suggest that the teacher establish a "secret" hand cue with your youngster—touching her nose or pulling her ear—to silently remind.

- **Simplify assignments**
  Ask the teacher to break all long-range assignments and instructions into smaller components. Let your child with TS do ten problems, rather than twenty; turn in a two-page composition, rather than eight pages and supplement oral instructions with a one-page written summary.

- **Verify written homework assignments**
  Ask the teacher to encourage your child to write down each homework assignment as it's given, then sign the sheet before the youngster leaves school. That helps you to know that the work being done is actually what was assigned for homework (and that, indeed, there actually was some homework assigned.) Some children prefer to tape the homework assignment. Some teachers also print assignments out each day and hand it to the youngster as he leaves class.

- **Allow extra time**
  If the teacher will agree to give your child extra time to complete a test or in-class assignment, she'll help him to compensate for the time lost to distractions, tics, and other difficulties. If other students complain about unfair advantage, remind them that everyone is different and that some students need different accommodations depending on their need.

- **Be aware of medication side effects**

The medications used to treat TS as well as its associated disorders work because they change the chemical balance in the brain. But they sometimes also create unwanted side effects that teachers may notice before parents do. Communicate often with your child's teachers, especially when medications have been changed or dosages altered. Then, when the teacher sees inattention and daydreaming, he'll know that these "driftings" could actually be the effect of the powerful drugs.

Some of these medications also may interfere with a child's cognitive processes, especially short-term memory. Others may make a child drowsy, enough to fall asleep in class. Still others may trigger depression. Obviously, these and other side effects make it difficult for a youngster to remain alert, focused, and on task. They also may cause social repercussions.

- **Be creative**

One of my children with TS had such a severe head jerk that he kept losing his place in the book when he tried to read. I took a piece of cardboard and cut a narrow rectangle out of it so that he could cover all but the lines he was reading.

If your child's tics are so bad that he cannot write or it takes too long to even take notes, ask the administration to let him use a laptop in class. If the school system cannot provide this aid, try to find a business to either donate its older laptops or perhaps, even buy the child a new one.

If your child is easily distracted, request that he take untimed tests in the library or school office. If the tics are so bad that he has difficulty writing, ask if he can take oral tests.

Suggest that teachers create a secret signal between them and the child with tics so he can leave the classroom when it's difficult to hold tics in. It's better for the child and better for the classmates.

You may hesitate to request special privileges for your child, but it's really no different than other accommodations made for children with visual or auditory handicaps, diabetes, etc. The purpose of school is for children to learn and, in order to learn, some children require accommodations. Hopefully, your child's teachers and administration are willing to be creative in ways that help your child achieve success in school.

Don't Rule Out College In Your Child's Future

Never assume that having TS prevents your child from achieving a college education. There are many, many adults with TS who have earned degrees, not only from college, but also from advanced programs. They have become physicians, lawyers, accountants, scientists, engineers, actors, writers, etc.

If your young adult has associated conditions, such as obsessive compulsive disorder and/or attention deficit disorder, some of the same accommodations that brought success in high school may also be needed in order to enjoy achievement in college.

- **Determine what type of college atmosphere is the best fit**

You and your youngster should meet with the high school college counselor during the junior year to discuss the pros and cons of college size and location. A large college or university offers more diversity which means your child probably will find a greater number of people who have a variety of disabilities. Although many of the classes may be large, there also may be more variety of class offerings. However, the student with TS might feel lost being one of so many others.

A smaller school, on the other hand, may be able to give your child more personalized attention. Classes, while limited in variety, may be smaller and the professors more accessible.

Encourage your child to tell the college advisor what subjects or majors are of interest, taking into consideration that most kids change their majors at least once or twice during their college years. What about other activities? Many kids with TS play sports and find that the exercise often reduces the severity of their tics. Others find the same results performing on stage or in the orchestra or band. Intense focus seems to reduce symptoms in many people. Also, by college age, unless they're tired or under stress many with TS find that their tics have diminished.

Another option for young adults with severe tics who want to attend college, but are sensitive about it, is to investigate on-line classes. NOTE: Many of these on-line "schools" are not accredited, so do your research before enrolling. Once comfortable with the pace of studying, a young adult may develop enough self confidence to try a community college, and then a four-year college or university.

- **What about Housing?**

Most colleges and universities offer a variety of housing alternatives. Your young adult needs to consider whether he wants a private room or apartment so he doesn't bother others with his tics or prefers a roommate who, hopefully, will be understanding and interested in learning about TS.

- **Visit potential schools**

Take your young adult to visit a few of the schools suggested by the college counselor. This will give her an idea of what to expect, what a variety of campuses are like, and which feels more comfortable—a small college town atmosphere or a large city. Go with her, as kids, especially those with OCD or ADD, often don't remember all that's being said by the admissions people.

Once your child is accepted, visit the school disability office to learn what services are available. Do they offer a separate room and/or extra time for exams? If writing is a problem (as it is with many people with TS), can the student take an oral exam instead of a written one? If your child is still on meds that make her sleepy, ask if it possible to take a lighter course load? What medical facilities are available for students?

Often the college assigns another student to host visiting high school youngsters. Be sure your child asks about the activities on campus because social life is such an important part of the college experience.

Part Two:

It's All in the Family

Chapter 5

Coping with Sibling Reactions

There's no doubt that it's tough on siblings when a brother or sister has a chronic condition. Parents spend time taking that child to doctors to adjust medications, talking to teachers at school, constantly explaining the manifestations of TS, and worrying. The siblings are told to be understanding, even when their brother or sister has vocalizations or has major motor tics at church or synagogue, in the movies, or at school. They see peers teasing their sibling and feel as though they need to rush in to defend (and most of them will), although sometimes what they'd like to do is just walk away and pretend they didn't notice. It's frustrating, and they often feel as though their parents love the child with TS more. One sibling, now an adult, recalled, "It was so embarrassing when my brother made barking and hooting sounds. I just wanted to crawl into a hole and disappear. I love him, but it was hard not to resent him at times."

A girl who had more than one sibling with TS said, "I was the forgotten child. At times I wished I had TS, too."

What Can Parents Do to Help?
Try to understand what your non-TS child feels. It isn't really jealousy or sibling rivalry. It's more a feeling that because he doesn't have TS, he's not worthy of your attention. You may have inadvertently given that child more chores than the sibling

with TS or blamed him for starting squabbles between the siblings when, in truth, the arguments were just as often started by the child with TS.

By the way, these problems aren't unique. They happen in every home where there are children with a chronic condition. Even in a home where the child with TS is an only child, parents tend to give in and take over chores and responsibilities that rightfully should be delegated to the child.

How to Balance Your Attention

First of all, realize that it can't be done. At times, that teeter-totter is going to be somewhat unbalanced simply because your child with TS does have special needs that must be addressed and they are time consuming. You have appointments with the physician to alter or change the medication, meetings with teachers and coaches, and perhaps, visits with occupational therapists or psychologists. However, there are some things you can do to try to let your other children know that you love them as much and want to be with them too.

- Try to take some time alone with your non-TS children. Go shopping, have lunch together, or see a special movie.
- Let them know that you understand it is often difficult for them. Acknowledge that the constant sound of the vocalizations tires you, too.
- Listen to what your children are saying. Often, it's a big help for them just to be able to express how they feel and to know that you understand and care.
- Be sure to know who their friends are and where they go.
- Let them know what types of behavior are not permitted. Draw a line in the sand against teasing about the tics.

- Don't insist that they always include their sibling when they get together with their own friends.
- Do plan some regular family activities so they realize that their sibling with TS is more than just someone with tics. Picnics, board games, touch football games, etc. are just a few family activities to create memories for all your children.

Chapter 6

Deciphering Tics from Behavioral Issues

Many parents ask, "How do you distinguish between your child's tic and a behavioral problem?" Sometimes it can be confusing. Did your child purposely hit his sister or did a motor tic cause his arm to fly up? Does your daughter refuse to wear her wool school skirt because she's being stubborn or does she really have a tactile sensitivity, a sensation of discomfort with the feel of certain fabrics? Is your son making clucking sounds to irritate his siblings or can't he help it? The best way to know is to ask. In our experience, the child usually is honest, but also embarrassed, so accept the answer and don't make a big production out of it.

Remember, though, that all kids try to play one parent against the other from time to time. Kids with TS are no different. Parents may argue with one another with one believing the behavior is just the child's tics while the other is sure the youngster is acting up. At times, it's difficult to know for sure which is the truth because the tics wax and wane, causing the problem to change, and sometimes even overnight. Just about the time you and the rest of the family have gotten used to a specific tic or tics, they either go away or, more likely, they change, sometimes appearing in a more troublesome form than before.

Because you may feel guilty or you're trying to compensate for the teasing your child with TS may be experiencing, you might be tempted to make excuses and let him off the hook, concerning chores and other responsibilities. Don't. Siblings will resent it, and you'll not be doing your child with TS any favor. He or she feels different enough because of the tics. Don't make your child feel that he can get by with purposeful bad behavior or getting out of chores because you don't think he's capable or up to the task of making the bed, emptying the dishwasher, walking the dog, etc.

Chapter 7

Balancing Tics and Treatment

Once you know there's medication that can reduce the intensity of the tics, it's tempting to want your child to have sufficient medication so that the symptoms go away completely. But experts suggest that you strive only to minimize the severity of the tics, rather than eliminating them altogether. Consider how severe the symptoms are, whether or not your child is bothered by them, and if they are creating problems in school, work, and social interactions. Sometimes, we parents are bothered far more by the symptoms than our children are. We may push for medication for our child with TS when it may not be necessary. Remember that although these medications may be able to reduce symptoms, they also are powerful drugs and as such, have side effects that must be taken into consideration.

Also, most cases of Tourette Syndrome are mild, and don't ever require the use of medications. In fact, many people with TS never are diagnosed because they view their tics as "habits" or "allergies" and are not too bothered by them.

Find a Knowledgeable Clinician
All physicians, nurse practitioners, and psychologists may not have equal knowledge when it comes to understanding the many medications used for treating TS. You need to select a

clinician who is experienced in treating children with TS , has the time to monitor the effects of the drug as dosages usually need to be titrated (raised or lowered) for the best benefit with the least troublesome side effects. This professional should be someone with whom you and your child are comfortable. The doctor/patient relationship is very important as the tics tend to wax and wane and patience is needed by all. Numerous studies have shown that a patient is more likely to be compliant (follow a doctor's instructions) if it seems that the physician is caring, compassionate, and can communicate effectively.

Ask yourself these questions:

- Does our physician make us feel comfortable?
- Does he listen when I describe symptoms, new tics, and difficulties with medications?
- Does she explain the meaning of confusing medical jargon?
- Does he/she explain potential side effects of medications so I can make an informed decision?
- Is our physician compassionate?
- Does our physician return phone calls in a timely manner?
- Can I reach our doctor by e-mail?
- Even though doctors have limited time to spend with each patient, do we feel as though we're not being rushed?

If you can answer "yes" to these questions, you probably have a positive relationship with your physician. If not, you might consider checking around your community to see if there's another knowledgeable physician that might be a better "fit" for you. It's important to feel at ease with your physician because you'll be part of the team for a long time.

Where Can You Find a Knowledgeable Clinician?

Great you say, but I don't know where to find someone who knows about TS, let alone the medications needed to reduce symptoms. Where do I go?

You can always call the Tourette Syndrome Association (1-888-4-Tourette) for a list of physicians from your state who are experienced in treating TS with medication. If you live near a university with a medical school, contact them to see whether they have a movement disorder clinic or department. It's also possible that your pediatrician or internist knows who in the area treats TS. There may be a specialist there. Remember, though, most people with TS do not require medication unless the symptoms are severe or there are co-occurring additional conditions that interfere seriously with daily life.

Which Medications Are Used in Treating TS?

A variety of medications are used in treating TS by suppressing or reducing tics, although this wasn't their original use. Some are called "neuroleptics" and are classified as major tranquilizers. Another group are alpha adrenergic agonists, marketed for high blood pressure control, but are also effective in reducing the severity of tics for some. As with all medications, there are side effects, some minor and some more serious. That's why you need to have a clinician who is expert in prescribing and regulating dosages. Most of these medications are in pill form, although some are available in patch form.

Almost all tic-suppressing medications should be introduced slowly to find the lowest, but most effective dosage. Never discontinue a medication abruptly as this can actually make tics worsen.

For more specific information, contact the TSA and ask for the brochure that is a guide to Tourette Syndrome medications.

Chapter 8

Recognizing Related Disorders

As if it weren't enough to have Tourette Syndrome, there are additional related problems that often tag along. Two of them include Obsessive-Compulsive Disorder (OCD) and Attention Deficit Disorder (ADD), with or without hyperactivity. If hyperactivity is a component, the disorder is known as Attention Deficit Hyperactivity Disorder or ADHD. It is believed that about half of those with TS have varying degrees of ADHD, and, as with TS, it affects more boys than girls.

Obsessive-Compulsive Disorder
According to the National Institute of Mental Health, "Obsessive-Compulsive Disorder (OCD), is an anxiety disorder, characterized by recurrent, unwanted thoughts (obsessions) and/or repetitive behaviors (compulsions). Typical obsessions include fear of germs or dirt, or a fear of being hurt or hurting someone. Examples of repetitive behaviors are washing the hands over and over again, counting, checking and rechecking, or constant cleaning, all of which are performed with the hope of preventing obsessive thoughts or making them go away. Performing these so-called 'rituals,' however, provides only temporary relief, and not performing them markedly increases anxiety."

Obviously, having to wash your hands many times for it to feel just right, or being over-concerned with symmetry like checking to be sure the window shades are all exactly the same height or that your shoes are lined up just so, or counting and recounting pencils in the drawer, or coins in your pocket can be very time consuming and may even take over one's life.

Homemakers with OCD have confessed that they are compulsive cleaners, scrubbing the same things many times, counting and recounting the towels in the linen closet, and even the extra rolls of toilet paper (and buying more if the "right" number isn't there.) But because no one is home to observe, they can often keep their exhausting secret.

School children with OCD may rewrite an essay or term paper over and over, trying to make it perfect. Unfortunately, they frequently miss the deadline and get an "F" on an otherwise superior paper. If they count words over and over or struggle with obsessive thoughts, they may not even hear the teacher's lecture. Their OCD can make them late for class and other activities and may bring ridicule from their peers. Experts say that it's often OCD and not tics that tend to make these individuals slow to mature socially. As adults, they also tend to have difficulties in making friends or having relationships.

It's often difficult to diagnose OCD in someone with TS because it's easy to rationalize that a child washes his/her hands constantly because of a tic, or lines up the shoes in the closet because of a tic.

Attention Deficit Hyperactivity Disorder
According to the National Institute of Mental Health, "the principal characteristics of ADHD are inattention, hyperactivity, and impulsivity…**Hyperactive** children always seem 'on the go' or constantly in motion. They dash around touching or playing with whatever is in sight, or talk incessantly…They squirm and fidget in their seats or roam around the room…**Impulsive** children seem unable to curb their immediate reactions or think before they act. They will

often blurt out inappropriate comments, display their emotions without restraint, and act without regard for the later consequences of their conduct…They may grab a toy from another child or hit when they're upset…Children who are **inattentive** have a hard time keeping their minds on any one thing for any length of time and may get bored with a task after only a few minutes…Homework is particularly hard for these children. They will forget to write down an assignment, or leave it at school…often becoming easily distracted by irrelevant sights and sounds, failing to pay attention to details and making careless mistakes, …completely losing or forgetting things like toys, or pencils, books, and tools needed for a task."

Combine these problems with the vocal and motor tics of TS and you can see why children with these "tag-along" disorders need significant support from their understanding parents, educated teachers, coaches, and others who work with them.

Other additional problems that may develop with those who have TS include sleep disturbances, learning difficulties, sudden temper tantrums, and, in lesser cases, self-injurious behavior such as hitting walls, head butting, cutting themselves, etc.

Please note that while few people with TS have all of these associated disorders, many with TS experience none of them other than the neurological symptoms of TS.

Chapter 9

Knowing What TS Isn't

As with any medical problems, especially those that are not particularly well-known, there are many myths and generalities that are more false than true. Perhaps you've heard some of them from well-meaning friends and relatives and are confused about what to believe. Let's take a look at some of them:

- Tourette Syndrome is NOT a mental disorder; it IS a neurobiological disorder of the central nervous system.
- TS does NOT appear only in specific ethnic cultures; it is found in ALL ethnic groups.
- TS is NOT a "cursing disease." Most people who have TS do NOT have coprolalia (uttering obscene or socially unacceptable words or phrases, a symptom which about 10 percent of those with TS do) nor is that aspect necessary in order to make the diagnosis.
- Everyone with TS does NOT have the same type of symptoms. There ARE similarities... such as blinking, neck jerking, sniffing, throat clearing, etc., although all of these may vary in severity and frequency.
- All doctors are NOT knowledgeable about TS and its treatment or, if they are, they may not stay abreast of recent research. To find the facts, contact the Tourette Syndrome Association, Inc. at 1-888-4-Tourette.

- Don't believe everything you see on television about TS. Usually only the most severe cases are depicted.
- Don't believe everything you read on the Internet either. Many individuals only post their own experiences (or that of a friend or relative) and there's a great deal of misinformation out there. Instead, look for the information posted by well-known hospitals or university clinics. The TSA web site (http://tsa-usa.org) has an extensive array of educational videos and DVDs, including treatment and management of TS and co-occuring conditions, hearing a teen talking about having TS, articles on how to handle bullies, what to tell the teacher, and other information.
- Although TS is a chronic disorder, it does NOT shorten a person's life.
- TS can NOT be diagnosed by a test; it IS diagnosed by taking a complete medical history, and by observation, although tics often may actually be suppressed in a doctor's office.
- People with TS can NOT stop ticcing, although the vocalizations and motor tics can be suppressed for a short time. When the pressure builds up, however, the individual must eventually express their symptoms.
- TS is NOT caused by poor parenting techniques.
- If you have TS, it does not prevent your playing sports, playing music, becoming a CPA, actor, athlete, salesman, or even a physician.

Chapter 10

Reducing Stress

No one can eliminate all stress in his life. In fact, some stress comes from positive events, such as winning an award, traveling or completing a book or painting. Other stress is created by negative occurrences such as losing a job, time pressures, having a child with a chronic disorder, or the death of a loved one. An imagined event or worry can trigger as much negative stress as the actual event itself.

That's why it's so important for all of us to learn to deal with stress in our lives because it builds up and can trigger mental and physical disorders ranging from digestive upsets, headaches, anxiety, and difficulty sleeping to high blood pressure, a weakened immune system, and depression. But for those with TS and their families, it's especially vital to deal with stress because it also can make existing tics more severe, which in turn, creates more stress for everyone in the family.

They're Watching You

Children learn ways to handle stress by observing how their parents cope. There's an old saying, "Children may close their ears to advice, but open their eyes to example." So remember that you're being watched and mimicked. Don't reach for an unwholesome "cure all" when your household gets particularly up-tight. Instead, share healthy ways you have learned (or are learning) to deal with stressful situations. Begin

44

by teaching your kids that stress is part of life; we just need to minimize its negative effects.

Recognize Some of the Signs of Stress

Stress isn't all bad; it helps us react quickly to jump out of the path of a speeding car, grab the baby before she falls out of the high chair, or act to put out a kitchen fire before it spreads. But uncontrolled stress can be harmful. That's why it's so important to recognize the signs of stress, because then you can begin to reduce it and teach your children as well.

The following are just a few of the signs of stress:
- Rapid heartbeat
- Aches in back, neck, shoulders, and stomach
- Fatigue
- Irritable bowel syndrome
- Procrastination/sense of futility
- Lack of appetite or eating too much
- Withdrawing
- Irritability
- Crying
- Depression
- Difficulty concentrating
- Forgetfulness
- Increase in symptoms for those with TS, OCD, ADD, and ADHD

Have a Schedule, but Build in Flexibility

This statement may seem at odds with itself, but what it means is that you lower stress when you have a definite schedule for your family so they know what's expected and when. It's even more important for you to build in some flexibility when your family has a child or children with TS. This is especially true if your youngster with TS also has ADD or OCD as well.

For example, if you're planning for a family outing at the movies, give the kids ample warning what time you all must be ready to get there in time. However, you also need to build in some flexibility in case your youngster with TS and ADD has to look for shoes, shirts, etc. If you don't have this "padding," the siblings in the car will start screaming for him/her to hurry up. Tension will build. The sibs will feel stressed, the parents will feel stressed, and the child who forgot what he was looking for, will definitely feel stressed, not remember where the shoes are, and start ticcing more intensely.

Learn and Practice the Relaxation Response
"The Relaxation Response" is a term created by Harvard Medical School cardiologist Herbert Benson, who literally wrote the book by the same title in 1975. Now Founder and President of the Mind/Body Medical Institute in Boston, Dr. Benson suggests using a combination of techniques for stress management, each of which will be discussed later in this chapter. The techniques are varied and include:

- Personal time
- Exercise
- Progressive relaxation
- Meditation
- Visualization
- Thought stopping
- Deep breathing
- Proper nutrition
- Yoga or Tai Chi
- Prayer
- Massage
- Connecting with others
- Joyful activities
- Laughter

Include a Personal Day For Yourself

This often is cited as the most difficult stress reduction technique to achieve when you have a child with TS who might also have associated behaviors. In addition, both parents may work, care for aging parents, juggle household chores and responsibilities with the other children, deal with behavioral problems and school issues. Where can you find a knowledgeable and qualified person to stay with your kids so you can have a brief, much needed respite? If only Mary Poppins would drop in to help.

Some parents use grandparents and extended family to spell them on occasion. Others trade off with other parents they've met through TS group meetings or their area's CH.A.D.D. (Children and Adults with Attention Deficit Disorder) chapter. Still others use students from nearby medical or nursing schools and in the process, help to educate these future medical professionals about these disorders.

Don't give up trying to find respite help. It's vital for you as individuals, your marriage, and, if you're a single parent, to revitalize you. You don't have to even be away over-night. Go out for lunch with a friend, shop, pamper yourself in a spa, stroll through a museum or art gallery. Everyone needs a vacation from constant responsibility. It not only will erase some of the stress you feel, but it also makes your child feel less dependent on you and helps develop self-confidence that others can help out too.

Try Exercise

Exercise is nature's tranquilizer; it improves cholesterol levels, lowers blood pressure, strengthens the immune system, boosts your metabolism, helps to keep weight in line, reduces stress, and also creates a sense of well-being. Fortunately, there isn't one "best" exercise; but there may be one or more than one that you enjoy and will do on a fairly regular basis. According to experts, any type of exercise is good as long as you like it so you'll do it often.

Walking is probably one of the easiest as it requires no special equipment, other than good shoes. Tics shouldn't interfere as they might with other types of exercise, so walking can become a family outing. If you don't enjoy walking, try biking (stationary or regular), boxing, rowing, skating (roller or ice), dancing, running, tennis, etc. **ALWAYS CHECK WITH YOUR PHYSICIAN BEFORE BEGINNING AN EXERCISE PROGRAM**, but once you have permission, try to exercise on a regular basis. Use exercise when you feel stressed and focus on how relaxation flows through your body.

Note: Don't use exercise as a competition or you'll just feel even more stressed.

Exercise is especially important for those with TS as it can somewhat reduce the severity and frequency of the tics by walking off excess energy. Although you might prefer to exercise alone, kids also enjoy this activity with their parents.

Practice Progressive Relaxation

Although many books make progressive relaxation sound complicated and mystical, it is neither. It simply is tensing and then relaxing your muscles one by one, from head to toe, so that you begin to recognize when your body feels tense. The theory is simple: If you're relaxed, you can't be tense. Just picture a cat sleeping on a table or window sill.

Follow these few steps and practice them about 15-20 minutes daily until you can relax your body more quickly:

1. Get comfortable on a bed or easy chair.
2. Breathe in deeply so your stomach rises as you breathe in, and falls as you exhale.
3. Tighten the muscles in your forehead, then relax while you breathe in deeply, and exhale.

4. Then work your way down from the muscles of your eyes, jaw, and neck through your arms and hands, chest, stomach, and pelvis, and down to your legs and toes.
5. Do a body check. You should feel more relaxed. Take a few more deep breaths.

You can find DVDs, tapes, and books describing this progressive muscle relaxation in more detail. Probably the best is still the original, *The Relaxation Response* by Herbert Benson, M.D.

Your children may be interested in learning this relaxation technique as well. Experts suggest that those with TS actually have fewer symptoms when they utilize relaxation techniques to reduce tension and fatigue. Many schools are using this type of stress training for their students. Relaxation is a life skill that everyone should use.

Meditation

Meditation, or what the Buddhists call "mindfulness" is an ancient art that teaches us to evoke the relaxation response. It has been used for centuries by Native Americans, religious leaders throughout the world, athletes, and theatrical performers. Meditation is the antithesis of multitasking as it teaches us to focus on just one thing, letting distractions fall by the wayside. Again, it isn't as complicated as you may think.

1. Get comfortable on your bed or an easy chair.
2. Focus on your breathing as before.
3. Empty your mind of extraneous thought and focus inward on a single word, such as "peace," "love," "God," or "Jesus."
4. If other thoughts pop into your head, return your focus to your breathing.

Some people focus on a flickering candle while others stare at a leaf, flower, or other object of nature.

Visualization

This is the relaxation technique that works best for me because I can take it with me. At first, you need to practice it, but it quickly becomes a technique you can call upon while you're standing in line at the check-out counter or are sitting in a doctor's waiting room. It's also an easy one to teach your kids.

1. Sit in a comfortable chair or lie on your bed.
2. Breathe in deeply and exhale as you did with the other exercises.
3. Picture a safe place that brings you joy, a place with happy memories.
4. Expand your senses so you can recall the scent, the sights, touch, and sound of that place.
5. When other thoughts invade your mind, ban them, and go back to the visualization of the picture you have created.

My "safe spot" is on a gentle sloping hill overlooking a bay filled with sailboats. I feel the warmth of the sun and the breeze against my cheeks. I hear the sound of the gulls overhead and smell the salt air from the bay below. As I begin to feel tension in my body I evoke this visualization whenever and wherever I am. I go to my "safe spot" before I go on TV or speak before an audience; I'm there when I go to bed and feel too stressed to fall asleep; I pay a quick visit when my date book is filled to over-flowing and I know I'm falling behind. Visualization always relaxes me.

Try it with your kids. You may be surprised to learn the spot they visualize as safe. It may be a real place filled with happy memories or a fictional one that they've created, but as long as going there relaxes them, it's working.

Thought Stopping

This relaxation technique is known in a number of different ways. Some call it "Affirmations," while others refer to it as "A

Mental Time Out" or "Cognitive Restructuring." The late Norman Vincent Peale called it "The Power of Positive Thinking." Actually, they all are pretty close to the same thing.

All of us have negative thoughts that pop into our head from time to time. "I feel fat," "I'm a failure as a parent," "I'll never get organized," "God must be punishing me with two kids with TS," or "My child is having difficulty in school so he'll never be able to go to college, hold a job, or have a family."

We have a choice to make when these negative thoughts pop into our head. We can agree with the thought and say, "Yes, I really AM a lousy parent" and "Yup, I'm sure God IS punishing me for something bad I've done." Or, we can push the thought stopping button in our head and say, "Stop" and then visualize our safe spot for a few minutes. It's faster than trying to rationalize with ourselves that we really aren't fat, a lousy parent, etc. It's quick, easy, and simpler than writing out affirmations (that we, in our negative state, may disagree with). Best of all, thought stopping also stops or at least slows the stress we're feeling from our negative thoughts.

Deep Breathing

You've read how to focus on deep breathing in some of the above relaxation techniques. It, in itself, is a type of meditation. Actors and singers call it "diaphragmatic breathing." As you take that deep breath, air coming in through your nose fills your lungs and makes your stomach rise. In the beginning, you might try putting a light weight book on your lower stomach so you can see that you're doing it correctly.

Concentrate on your breathing as your mind releases distracting thoughts. You breathe in, inhaling peace and tranquility and when you exhale, you release stress and anxiety. Use deep breathing as you wait for a red light to change, the grocery line to move, and when your child's TS or the siblings' squabbling make you feel stressed.

Proper Nutrition

Is eating a relaxation technique? It is when you stop gobbling your meals or eat standing up. Slow down. Take time to sit, put your napkin on your lap, and enjoy what you eat. You'll eat less because it takes 20 minutes from the time you begin eating for the brain to signal that you're full. What's more, your children will follow your pace and dinner time, especially, will become a family time, rather than a "gobble and go" experience.

Follow the 2005 United States Department of Agriculture's new "Food Pyramid" which has up to six ounces of whole-grain foods, at least 2 ½ cups of varied vegetables, and no more than two cups of a variety of fruits a day. Fish, poultry, and eggs should be eaten no more than two times a day and red meat, white rice, bread, potatoes, and sweets should be used only sparingly.

When you dine rather than dash, you'll eat less, have time to talk with your family, and feel less stressed. Let the kids help plan and prepare the menus. Once they learn about proper nutrition, they'll feel needed and involved.

Yoga, Tai Chi, and Qi Gong

Yoga has been practiced for centuries in India as a way to become more aware of your body and to elicit the relaxation response. It incorporates rhythmic breathing, meditation, and gentle stretching. You can usually find beginners' Yoga classes in community centers, spas, and some hospital programs. There are also DVDs and tapes, although it's probably better to work with an instructor who can give you pointers.

Like Yoga, Tai Chi also can help you slow down and relax through a series of specific motions. Qi Gong, an ancient

Chinese art, combines breathing, meditation, exercise, and flowing movements and it too, evokes the relaxation response. These three exercises focus the mind as they help you to reduce stress in your body.

The Power of Prayer

The mother of three children, all with TS, said she never found time to practice any of the above relaxation methods. "I just pray a lot," she said.

For some people prayers can be another form of relaxation. You fill your mind with the repetitive words learned in religious school as a child and, in doing so, you shut out the stresses of the outside world. Prayers offer comfort and a sense of peace to many.

If you and your family attend religious services, you join with others who can give you emotional support and, perhaps, even find those who could offer some respite care. In addition, many religious organizations have youth groups where youngsters can get together under supervision. This broadens the social network for your child and can even provide the leader of the congregation an opportunity to educate the other young people about understanding and learning tolerance of those who seem different.

Soothing Hands

Our family is a family of huggers. I still say to my husband, kids, or grandkids, "I need a hug." When my kids with TS had exhausting tics, I'd hold them or rub their back, arm, or neck and could almost feel the tension easing.

Years ago, Sherry Suib Cohen, co-author of *The Magic of Touching*, wrote some words I've quoted frequently. She said, "You can't give a touch without getting one right back. You can talk, listen, smell, see, and taste alone, but touch is a reciprocal act."

Massage is one such type of touch. I can personally vouch for the stress reducing attributes of massage as I've had the same massage therapist for 24 years and she often says, "You're holding tension in your back and that's what's affecting your neck," or "I feel a lot of tension in your forearm. What's doing?"

- Unless you're one of those people who doesn't like to be touched (and there are many), you can find a massage therapist in spas, beauty shops, hotels, and health clubs. You can also find qualified massage therapists through your closest medical school, rehabilitation facility, orthopedist, or possibly the physical education department of a college or university. If your state requires licensing, be sure your therapist is credentialed.

There are many different types of massage—Swedish, sports, Shiatsu, hot rocks, and deep tissue to name a few-- so don't try one and give up. You may have to experiment until you find the type of massage that relaxes you best. People also differ in whether or not they want background music so speak up. The massage therapist is not a mind reader.

Connecting with Others

We humans are social animals. We gain approval, emotional support, and energy from interacting with others. But parents with a child with TS often feel that they have no time for social activity. They're worn out, fatigued, and have no time left for what they consider "frivolities." But if that describes you, think again. You need to reach out to others who may think you want to be left alone and so they do just that. Call up a neighbor or someone you've met through your children's school, your community center, religious institution, or at a TSA meeting.

If you're shy about being with new people who don't understand what TS is, think of this as an opportunity to educate them. Let them meet your child and see his positives, so they understand that a person with TS is just that, an individual with many fine qualities, but who also has TS.

People fear the unknown. When they see a child making strange sounds and jerking movements, they often become fearful. They may be frightened that it's catching or that their child may be frightened. But learning even a little about the disorder and given the opportunity to get to know your youngster, those fears may quickly fly away.

Getting together with others for coffee, a neighborhood cookout, or a friendly game will relieve stress. You'll find your tension melting and enjoy yourself.

Joyful Activities

Doing more can actually reduce stress, especially if the "more" is fun, enjoyable, and makes you laugh. The activities can be something you enjoy doing alone such as sketching, painting, writing in a journal, etc. They can be done with a spouse or friend or with your entire family as long as it's fun. For some, that may be a fishing trip, camping, hiking, or learning to do line dancing or square dancing. For others, learning Chinese cooking, a new language, joining a choir, acting in a play, growing orchids, or even volunteering to help others in some way. Ralph Waldo Emerson said, "It is the most beautiful of compensations of this life that no man can try to help another without helping himself."

The activities should bring you pleasure, hold your focus so you relax and forget your stresses. This escape is your refueling mode, the vital need your body has in order to avoid burnout. Don't neglect yourself. Whether you have TS or members of your family do, this is a gift to yourself, a gift that also can be enjoyed by others.

Laughter

Although the quotation, "Laugh and the world laughs with you" is familiar to most people, the late Norman Cousins is often credited with the recent acceptance by lay and medical professionals alike of the healing power of laughter. A good laugh is the body's natural tranquillizer because it triggers the release of endorphins, which help the body reduce stress. Laughing makes you breathe more deeply, therefore bringing more air into your lungs. It also helps to lower blood pressure, reduce muscle tension, and to improve blood circulation. Laughter is what Norman Cousins called "inner jogging." What's more, it's something the entire family can do together.

Teach the kids to look for the funny side of life. Have a comedy night with funny DVDs and jokes. Laugh at your own foibles and show your kids that laughter has healing powers.

PART Three:

Adult Issues

Chapter 11

Getting a Job

Just as school is children's work, finding employment is adult's work. Often parents worry whether their children with TS will be able to find employment when they become adults. Sometimes, to prevent disappointment, they let adult children move back into their home and continue to financially support them. But this may be an unnecessary and unwise move. Be assured that people with Tourette Syndrome participate in all kinds of work—from artists, accountants, actors, and athletes, to cooks, computer programmers, and financial planners, lawyers, musicians, nurses, salespeople, teachers, technicians, physicians, social workers, writers, web designers, ventriloquists and veterinarians.

Childhood Problems May Be Assets in Adulthood

There's no doubt that the structure of most of our elementary, middle, and high schools work against children with TS, especially those with OCD and ADD or ADHD symptoms as well. But those negatives often become positives in adulthood when excess energies that once drove teachers crazy actually help the actor, salesperson, musician, or athlete. The distractibility and "different" way of looking at something can be harnessed in adult pursuits such as writing, art, music, technology, research, and film making. The late Carl Jung, a Swiss psychiatrist and psychologist, praised inattention, daydreaming, and risk-taking behavior by saying, "Without this playing with fantasy, no creative work has ever yet come to birth."

Adults, like Thomas Edison, who couldn't sit still in school and quickly dropped out, should take comfort in knowing that Edison's inability to concentrate on one subject for any length of time actually led him into greater experimentation.

How to Find the Right Job

Think about what you'd like to do. Don't reject possibilities just because of your symptoms. You want to find a job in which you can be successful, so it's important to take an honest look at the type and severity of your symptoms. Because stress and tension in trying to stick to deadlines or a rigid schedule trigger tic intensity for most people, most adults with TS suggest that you focus on employment offering flexibility But this is where you need to know yourself as everyone is unique.

One adult with TS and OCD advised, "Stay away from jobs where you have to follow specific orders, like the military." But another, also with TS and OCD, reported that his life in the military was ideal for him. "My OCD makes me the perfect officer," he said. "I do everything by the book."

Think carefully about what you enjoy doing and where. Do you like to work in the outdoors or in an office environment? Alone or with other people? With background music and noise or opt for little extra stimulation? Play to your strengths. If deadlines make your symptoms worse, think twice about working for an ad agency or news bureau. If you enjoy being your own boss, consider starting a small business. If you're too distracted to ever get organized, find employment where time limits are less important and you can focus on one task at a time.

If your tics are severe or you have coprolalia, (swearing or saying "dirty" or misappropriate words) think about an outside job such as a fishing guide, truck driver, or landscaper.

There's no doubt that finding a job that fits your particular needs as well as one you enjoy helps to reduce stress. This is important for everyone, regardless if he/she has TS or not. The hours you spend working, your co-workers, and the environment surrounding you all affect your personal well-being. Consider any potential employment carefully.

Although there are numerous books describing how to find the "perfect" job and interview for it, you might read one of the first and still best in its field, *What Color Is Your Parachute?* Written by Richard Nelson Bolles, and originally published in 1970, it is revised annually. Bolles and his co-author Dale Brown have also written *Job-Hunting for the So-Called Handicapped* which you also might want to read if your tics are particularly severe and you also have OCD and/or ADD. But remember what Bolles says should be your mantra: **"No matter what handicap you have, or think you have, it cannot possibly keep you from getting hired. It can only keep you from getting hired at *some places*."** Repeat that whenever you get discouraged.

Bolles also adds this realistic note: "As a disabled job-hunter, part of your task in job-hunting is that you will *often* have to educate would-be employers, as you go." But then, as someone with TS, you have been educating teachers, coaches, service people, neighbors, and friends for years so you're really an expert by now.

Where to Find Possible Jobs
While there are web sites, such as www.monster.com, www.craigslist.org, and www.CareerBuilder.com, according to Bolles, "Research has turned up the fact that out of every 100 job-hunters who use the Internet as their search method for finding jobs, 4 of them will get lucky and find a job, while 96 job-hunters out of the 100 will not---if they only use the Internet to search for a job."

There are also local temporary employment agencies where you can try out various types of jobs to test which ones feel comfortable. Let others know you are looking for work. "Who you know" may not get you a job, but others may open doors for an interview. One of my daughters got her first teaching job because a co-worker at her temporary job with a building company said his mother, an elementary school principal, was interviewing teachers. She made the call, got the interview, was hired, and worked for eight years at that same school.

If you go to an employment agency, be sure you understand who pays the fee. It may be the employer, but if it's you, the fee will be taken out of your paycheck.

You also can read about potential jobs in the newspaper's want ad section, but a good way to find a job is to hear about it from a friend as many jobs are filled even before they are posted. That's why you need to tell everyone you know that you're looking for a job and provide specifics about the job you'd like to find.

Once you hear about something that might be a good fit, immediately contact the human relations department and ask for an appointment. Don't just send in your resume and hope for the best. And don't procrastinate. Those who wait to make a move, lose out. (The early bird...and all that).

Not Your Grandparents' Office
When you think about working in an office, forget about the stereotypical office with rows of desks and with the proverbial water cooler down the hall. That was yesterday's offices for the most part. Today many are virtual offices housed in your car, boat, home, or even the closest coffee shop.

According to communication consultant Andy Shimberg (yes, my son) suggests that "the perfect virtual office has a laptop computer, access to the Internet using both a WIFI card in the notebook and a cellular modem (so you don't need to be at a hotspot). You'd have an Efax number (which gives you incoming/outgoing fax capability through the Internet) and probably use a social networking site like Linked In or Facebook for your online Rolodex. If you're really advanced, you'll probably write a Blog and participate in a number of Wikis, depending on what your personal hobbies or business interests were."

If you understand the above paragraph (which I do not), you probably could be successful working in a virtual office. If it really is Greek to you, find a fantastic mentor to help educate you or stick to a more traditional office experience. But there are many types of jobs where you can work at home or even on a shared basis, such as handling bookkeeping chores for small businesses, tutoring students, programming, or, in the case of job sharing, teaching half a day and have someone else teach the other half.

Know Your Employment Rights
It's important for you to know about the legal protections guaranteed by Federal Law for anyone with a handicap. Section 504 of the Rehabilitation Act of 1973 provides that "no otherwise qualified individual with handicaps in the United States…shall, solely by reason of …handicap, be excluded from the participation in, be denied benefits of, or be subjected to discrimination under any program or activity receiving Federal financial assistance."

But the Americans with Disabilities Act of 1990 (ADA) went further, eliminating discrimination in all areas, not just those federally funded. The ADA makes it illegal to discriminate in employment against a qualified individual with a disability. Obviously, the operative word is *qualified*. If you have the ability, education, and training to do a particular job, and your qualifications are superior to others also applying for the position, you cannot be denied employment because you have TS.

The ADA states, "An employer is required to provide reasonable accommodation to a qualified applicant or employee with a disability *unless* (my italics) the employer can show that the accommodation would be an undue hardship… that is, would require significant difficulty or expense."

The reality of this is that the employer would have to accommodate your symptoms by moving your desk so your arm tic wouldn't cause you to clobber your co-worker; rearrange your work table so it would face inward, rather than toward a window, another employee, or other distracting view; or allow you to use a computer if your motor tics caused your handwriting to be illegible.

"Your employer would not, however, have to build you a special soundproof office if your vocal tics made it difficult for other employees to perform their work."[1]

Don't be afraid to ask for accommodations if you require them. Most workers have them in some way. As a southpaw, I always have to move the telephone to the right side of the desk so I can use my left hand to write. (I also need a step-stool to reach high bookshelves because I am vertically challenged.) Others may have an attachment on their phone so they can hear more clearly or have manuals with larger than standard print.

To Tell or Not to Tell
People whose tics are fairly minor have asked whether or not they should tell a prospective employer that they have TS. The vote is somewhat split, although the majority seem to feel that "honesty is the best policy." That response may be bolstered by

---

[1] Shimberg, Elaine Fantle, *Living with Tourette Syndrome* (New York, Fireside, Simon & Schuster) 1995, p192-3

the fact that the Americans with Disabilities Act (ADA) makes it illegal to refuse to hire a **qualified** person based on his/her disability. As you'll note, *qualified* is the operative word.

If you do tell, have an information sheet with questions the prospective employer might have along with your answers as to how you could handle a particular problem. Be open and matter of fact. Keep it simple and don't over-explain. Focus instead on what you *can* do, rather than what you cannot, and have references in hand. Always mention what accommodations you'll need, such as short breaks if you feel the tics building up.

The 10 Commandments of Job Interviewing

1. *Do your homework so you know what the company does.*
2. *Update your resume to show how you could fit in.*
3. *Be on time; arrive early so you can relax and collect your thoughts.*
4. *Dress professionally.*
5. *No gum chewing.*
6. *Think before you speak.*
7. *Be honest. Don't give yourself fake credentials and degrees.*
8. *Ask questions that show you know something about what the company does.*
9. *Have confidence in what you can do.*
10. *Write a thank you note regardless of whether you get the job or not; they may know someone else who can use a bright, polite, and capable person such as you.*

Chapter 12

Dating

(For adults with TS)

The "D" word is unnerving to many adults with Tourette Syndrome. Their adolescence, a time that is difficult at best for most youngsters, may have been even more troublesome for them because that's when their tics were at their worst. In case you've forgotten, teenagers are not known for being supportive of those who seem "different." While peers were going to parties, proms, and plays, many teens with TS remained on the sidelines. Their experiences relating to others, making friends, dating, and first love were slim, to say the least.

Even if your tics have lessened by adulthood, those scars remain. Even though you may identify with those youthful memories, don't feel that you still need to remain on the bench. You are grown-up now, and it's time for you to become a player. Just make sure that you pick the right game and the right teammates.

Look for Friendships First
There's no doubt that stress usually make tics worse, so the best idea is to find a playing field where you feel comfortable. Don't focus on finding someone to date right away. Instead, engage in activities that you enjoy such as volunteer work, study groups, going to museums and art galleries, taking a class

in pottery or oil painting, learning a new language, or joining a gym. The people you meet will be there for the same reason that you are. They enjoy it.

Introduce yourself and talk about your interests. Ask what the other person likes to do. Then, perhaps, you both can go out for coffee as friends. If you still have tics and they're noticeable or you're showing obvious symptoms of OCD, explain that you have TS with some OC behaviors and unless the other person asks questions, drop it. Listen, more than you talk. Hopefully, you'll find yourself relaxing and enjoying this friendship.

Unfortunately, it often is the behavioral problem, not the TS symptoms, that interferes in a relationship. Try to find humor and be honest about your frustration in not being able to control certain behaviors, and hope that those you meet will understand. Actually, you may even learn that some of them admit to having "a little" OCD themselves.

Support Groups Can be Helpful

C.S. Lewis, an English novelist and essayist, said it best. "Friendship is born at the moment when one person says to another, 'What! You too? I thought I was the only one." That is the theory behind support groups of all kinds. They help you realize that you're not alone.

TSA support groups, can also help you strengthen your self-image, relax more, and make new friends. Others who have experienced the same difficulties during adolescence as you have can describe how they've overcome behavior problems, learned to listen, become less judgmental of others, and how they've gained control of impulsivity, tantrums, and distractibility. Those who lose their temper easily because they have to stand in a line, for example, can describe useful avoidance techniques, such as going shopping on a quieter time of day rather than the noon hour, or midweek rather than on Friday. They also can share their own techniques for defusing rages such as having a punching bag at home or exercising to blow off steam.

Carolyn R. Shaffer and Kristin Anundsen, co-authors of *Creating Community Anywhere: Finding Support and Connection in a Fragmented World* write, "support groups allow you to be yourself, to tell the truth about both your weaknesses and your strengths…"

The only caveat about support groups is to be sure that they don't turn into gripe sessions where you leave feeling more depressed than when you arrived.

Where to Find Potential Dates

Despite what you might think, there are people everywhere who are wondering the same thing. It's a matter of you both being in the same place at the same time. So, rather than sitting home and wishing you could find someone to be with, go to where people are.

You may immediately think of a bar. It's noisy, and no one can hear your tics; it's dark, so no one can see them either. The only problem is that in a bar it's so noisy and dark that you can't hear what anyone is saying and this may be important. Do you really want to meet people who hang out in bars?

- Go somewhere new, such as an antique exhibit, flower show, dog show, or museum. Smile at others and you'll usually see them smile or at least nod back at you.
- Find a new activity—hockey, basketball, bowling, softball, soccer, etc. You'll find fans who can explain the rules and if you try playing, you may surprise yourself that while you're focusing, your tics are not that noticeable.

- Look for announcements for book clubs, hobby clubs, and other activities. Your community center, local college or university, or religious organization may sponsor study groups, play-reading groups, etc. where you'll find others who share your interests.
- Change single groups. If you've been going to the same single-mingles, branch out and try another so you can meet new and different people. Even if you don't meet anyone you enjoy going out with, someone there may know someone whom they'd love to fix you up with.
- Join a gym so you'll not only get a good workout, but you'll also meet new people who enjoy exercise.
- Take that class you've always wanted to take. Community colleges and YMCAs offer everything from pottery to poetry.
- Volunteer. You'll help others and find other volunteers who have the same interests as you do. What's more, when you volunteer, you stop thinking about yourself and begin to think of the others you're making happy.

Stop Looking for the Perfect Person

None of us is perfect, but many people still expect perfection in the other person. In my book, *Another Chance for Love*, co-authored with Sol Gordon, Ph.D., we wrote about Clara, a lonely woman who was depressed and had no friends. At her therapist's suggestion, she began working at a home for abused children and before long, she felt needed, wanted, and appreciated.

But something else happened. Clara met another volunteer there, a short, bald man. She admitted thinking he was "kind of ugly." But they quickly became friends through their work and she looked forward to seeing him. It occurred to her after a few months, that she couldn't understand why she had thought he was ugly. Instead, she had looked beyond his outward appearance and found a wonderful friend.

Stop looking at another's imperfections. Everyone (including you) has them. The "myth model" doesn't exist and you're missing a lot of pleasure in life if you wait to find the perfect person.

Practice these 10 things to feel good about yourself:
1. *Develop a sense of humor (but never use it to be hurtful)*
2. *Smile at others*
3. *Listen more than you speak*
4. *Accept what you can't change*
5. *Help others through volunteerism*
6. *Bounce back from disappointments*
7. *Be open to learning new things*
8. *Praise others so they can feel good about themselves*
9. *Think about your special gifts; everyone has them*
10. *Believe in yourself*

If you've ever had a golf lesson, you know that instructors say, "Don't look at the ball; look at where you want it to go." The same is true for how each of us should live our lives: look towards where we want to go and trust that happiness and success will follow.

My grandmother used to say, "Everyone (even those without TS) has something." This is what you have (as do so many others), so never crawl into a cave and hide from others. Learn to laugh at your foibles and ease up on yourself. That opens you up to real friendships with others. By looking for friendship first, you give yourself breathing space to gain confidence and strengthen your self-esteem. You are a special person. You're bright, have a good sense of humor, and are interesting, so shut the door on those emotional painful childhood memories. Welcome to the new world of adults.

Chapter 13

Securing Housing

This may seem like an unusual chapter in a book about TS, but it's an important one for those who have vocal tics that may be annoying to others. In a Catch 22 scenario, often young adults with troubling vocal tics may find it difficult to secure a job and without work, there is no income. As with many young adults even without TS, the answer sometimes is going home to Mother and Dad. And the parents of those with TS, knowing the rejection their child has experienced over the years, quickly lay down the welcome mat.

Give Your Adult Children Wings
But just as Mommy Bird knows when it's time to push the little ones out of the nest, it's important for us to encourage our adult children, especially those with TS, to find homes of their own. It tells them that we have confidence in them and trust their ability to "fly" on their own, and that although we will always love and support them, we cannot protect them from life as an adult.

When we close ranks, bringing our adult child into the castle and raising the drawbridge, protecting them from the harshness of the outside world, we're subtly telling them that we don't think they can make it on their own. According to pediatric psychologist James Kenneth Whitt, "Feelings of vulnerability and inadequacy may become self-fulfilling if, paradoxically, the child withdraws from developmental contention and sustains (or even provokes) interpersonal rejection in order to maintain the now internalized identity as a vulnerable, crippled, socially abandoned person who must depend on close family members for needed care."[2]

Dr. Whitt suggests that parents can help an adult child by what he calls "practice sessions." That means asking them questions that pose problems or difficulties for an adult with TS in order to garnish positive responses or at least, get the individual to think about what they could/should be. Such questions might be, "What will you tell a prospective landlord about your tics?" or "How will you tell your new neighbors why you sometimes hoot, bark, or say inappropriate things?"

What to Look For in Housing
Obviously, cost is important, even when parents help supplement the rent for a time. If your adult child doesn't drive, it's vital that the housing unit is close to public transportation.

A major consideration for someone with loud vocal tics, of course, is sound proofing, a condition greatly lacking in rental units, condos (even expensive ones), or town-houses (often known as "town-homes"). You usually can hear toilets flushing and showers running because the plumbing pipes are usually stacked. You may hear babies crying, neighbors fighting (or making love), and televisions and sound systems blaring.

You might consider your housing in a neighborhood that borders on being commercial so that the street sounds mask your vocal tics. If possible, look for an end unit, and make your bedroom the one with a common wall to your neighbor as most people with TS have fewer, if any, tics while they sleep. Use

---

[2] Whitt, James Kenneth, "Children's Adaptation to Chronic Illness and Handicapping Conditions." *Chronic Illness and Disability Though the Life Span*, Springer Publishing Company, New York, 1984.

carpeting, heavy drapes, and upholstered furniture whenever possible to help absorb sounds.

Meet your Neighbors

Do take time to meet your neighbors and tell them you have TS, explaining what that means. That way, they won't be surprised if they hear sounds when you're washing your car, walking the dog, getting the mail, sunbathing or using your grill.

If you don't feel comfortable describing TS face-to-face with the people next door, write them a note, introducing yourself and sharing a little about your symptoms. That may erase the fear most people have about someone who acts differently, especially in today's society when we all might worry about strangers who may be on drugs, drunk, or are just plain weird.

Include in your friendly introduction the people you'll do business with in this new neighborhood, folks like the mail person, bank personnel, dry cleaners, grocery and drug store clerks, health club, hair stylist, etc. If you feel uncomfortable doing this, type up a one-page "Q&A" about TS and hand it to them. This shows them that you are intelligent, emotionally in control, and a potentially good customer for them, even though you have a neurological condition.

This may seem like overkill, but I heard of a young man with TS who had coprolalia. He joined a new health club and soon found himself confronted by an angry African American gentleman who had taken exception to his unfortunate vocal tic, a racial slur. When the young man introduced himself and explained that he had TS and couldn't control this objectionable vocal tic, the man was understanding and they actually became good friends. That's why it's important to make the effort to educate people before they have a chance to react negatively.

Chapter 14

Looking into the Future

What is the future for someone with Tourette Syndrome? Actually, it's very promising.

Fortunately, many children with TS find that their tics dissipate considerably as they pass through adolescence into their adult years. Hopefully, self-confidence hasn't been totally shaken during those difficult years of being teased and perhaps even bullied by youthful peers. Those who do have emotional or self-image problems, however, can often be helped through counseling sessions with qualified therapists.

Although many adults no longer have the tics that plagued them so in childhood, many still have a few hints of tics when they are over-tired or under a great deal of stress. (That's all the more reason to get plenty of sleep and to learn and practice the stress reduction techniques detailed in Chapter 10.)

Also, new technologies are emerging that will change many things in the TS world. Even today, biofeedback is being explored as a possible non-medical treatment for tics. Improved imaging techniques now allow researchers to view the brain and observe how it functions in those with TS.

Tourette Syndrome Has Come Out of the Shadows
Thanks to the work of the national Tourette Syndrome Association, Inc., more people are learning the truth about what

TS really is. The previous distortions of fact in television shows, presenting actual falsehoods about the disorder or only illustrating the worst case scenarios, have given way to positive programs like the TSA/HBO Emmy Award winning documentary, "I Have Tourette's but Tourette's Doesn't Have Me."

Joining forces in 2005, The Centers for Disease Control and Prevention (CDC) and the Tourette Syndrome Association educated well over 15,000 professionals in medicine, nursing, psychology, social work, education, and other disciplines by 2007. Special "Physicians Training Retreats" organized by the TSA, educate physicians throughout the U.S. Once having completed such a program, the physicians may be included on TSA physician referral list. Other programs are offered to educators, not only teaching them about TS, but also offering suggestions on how to handle the tics, outbursts, learning disabilities, etc. within the classroom and on the athletic fields.

Yes, Tourette Syndrome is no longer languishing in the shadows, a victim of mystery and myths. Although there as yet is no cure, education has increased understanding and acceptance.

RESOURCES

Tourette Syndrome Association, Inc.
42-40 Bell Blvd. Suite 205
Bayside, NY 11361-2820
(718) 224-2999
Fax: (718) 279-9596
http://tsa-usa.org

Children and Adults with Attention Deficit Disorders
CHADD
800-233-4050
8181 Professional Place #150
Landover, MD 20785
(301) 306-7070
Fax: (301) 306-7090
www.chadd.org

OC FOUNDATION
Info@ocfoundation.org
P.O. Box 961029
Boston, MA 02196
(617) 973-5801
Fax: (617) 973-5082

Learning Disabilities Association of America
4156 Library Road
Pittsburgh, PA 15234-1349
(412) 341-1515
Fax: (412) 344-0224

SUGGESTED READING

Baskin, Amy and Fawcett, Heather. *More Than a Mom: Living a Full and Balanced Life When Your Child Has Special Needs* (Rockville, MD: Woodbine House, 2006)

Berecz, John M. Ph.D. *Understanding Tourette Syndrome, Obsessive Compulsive Disorders & Related Problems* (New York: Springer Publishing Company, 1992)

Bruun, Ruth Dowling and Bruun, Bertel. *A Mind of Its Own: Tourette Syndrome: A Story and a Guide.* (New York and Oxford: Oxford University Press, 1994)

Campito, Jan Starr. *Supportive Parenting: Becoming an Advocate for Your Child with Special Needs* (London and Philadelphia: Jessica Kingsley Publishers, 2007)

Chowdhury, Uttom. *Tics and Tourette Syndrome* (London: Jessica Kingsley Publishers, 2004)

Chowdhury, Uttom and Robertson, Mary M.D. *Why Do You Do That? A Book About Tourette Syndrome for Children and Young People* (London: Jessica Kingsley Publishers, 2006)

Fields, Evelyn M. *Bully Blocking: Six Secrets to Help Children Deal with Teasing and Bullying* (London and Philadelphia: Jessica Kingsley Publishers, 2007)

Hartmann, Thom, *Attention Deficit Disorder: A Different Perception* (Lancaster, Pennsylvania: Underwood-Miller, 1993)

Hallowell, Edward M., M.D. and Ratey, John J., M.D. *Driven to Distraction: Recognizing and Coping with Attention Deficit Disorder from Childhood through Adulthood* (New York: Simon & Schuster, 1994)

Heininger, Janet E. Ph.D., and Weiss, Sharon K., M.Ed. *From Chaos to Calm* (New York: Perigee Books, 2001)

*Krueger, Tira, illustrated by Dineen, Tom, *Taking Tourette Syndrome to School* (Plainview, NY: JayJo Books, 2001)

McNamara, Barry E., Ed.D., and McNamara, Francine J., M.S.W., C.S.W. *Keys to Parenting a Child with Attention Deficit Disorder* (Hauppauge, NY: Barron's Educational Series, Inc., 1993)

Marsh, Tracy Lynne, *Children with Tourette Syndrome: A Parents' Guide* (Rockville, MD: Woodbine House, 2007)

*Noner, Holly L., illustrated by Treatmer. Meryl, *I Can't Stop! A Story about Tourette Syndrome* (Morton Grove, Illinois: Albert Whitman & Company, 2005)

Seligman, Adam Ward & Hilkevich, John S. *Don't Think About Monkeys* (Duarte, CA: Hope Press, 1992)

Shimberg, Elaine Fantle, *Living with Tourette Syndrome* (New York: Fireside, Simon & Schuster, 1995)

Weiss, Gabrielle and Hechtman, Lily Trokenberg *Hyperactive Children Grown Up* (New York: The Guilford Press, 1993)

Weiss, Dr. Lynn, *Attention Deficit Disorder in Adults* (Dallas: Taylor Publishing Company, 1992)

Zarzour, Kim, *Facing the Schoolyard Bully* (Buffalo, NY: Firefly Books, 2000)

*Starred books are for children

Index